Vitality

Vitality

YOUR BODY

LOVES YOU,

LOVE IT BACK

Celeste Reese Willis, MD

MOUNTAIN ARBOR PRESS

MOUNTAIN ARBOR
PRESS
Alpharetta, GA

ISBN: 978-1-63183-809-5 - Paperback
eISBN: 978-1-63183-810-1 - ePub
eISBN: 978-1-63183-811-8 - mobi

Library of Congress Control Number: 2020903790

Printed in the United States of America   0 2 2 5 2 0

♾This paper meets the requirements of ANSI/NISO Z39.48-1992 (Permanence of Paper)

This book is dedicated to my mother, Betty W. Reese. Your unwavering support and encouragement along my untraditional journey through medicine has meant more than you can imagine. Thank you for teaching me that the prayers of a mother, on behalf of her child, will be answered by God no matter the situation nor circumstance. I would not be where I am today without your love and support. Thank you for blessing me with the amazing benefit of a praying mother.

I also dedicate this book to my father, James Reese Jr. Thank you for every five a.m. wakeup call on the days we had tests from elementary school through high school. You taught me at an early age the importance of investments. Investment into my education would be the leading tool, with God being there in every way to turn to on the hardest days. Thank you instilling the love of family into me. Thank you.

This book is also dedicated to my loving husband, Vincent Willis Jr. Thank you for your unwavering support throughout this entire process. It is such a blessing to have someone who wants to see me win as my partner, best friend, and husband. You have been patient, supportive, encouraging, giving, and loving to me during this entire process. I never thought I could love you more than on our wedding day, and yet here it is. I love you.

CONTENTS

PREFACE

I, Celeste Reese Willis, MD, help busy professionals through virtual medicine, direct primary care, and concierge medicine visits that allows them to continue to live their best, while I assess and aid them in finding solutions to their acute and general medical care needs. I help keep the healthy professional lively and vigorous.

As a young child, I was initially exposed to the field of medicine via a shadowing program with my high school. When I later matriculated through medical school, I watched my mother suffer from the complications of Coronary Artery Disease. As I began to learn about medicine, my later teachings were filtered through those experiences. I easily saw the benefit of how prevention can impact a person's life. Continuing through residency, I began to moonlight at an urgent care center. After trying traditional medicine for three years, I went back to urgent care medicine due to my love of the acuity and efforts of being able to quickly enhance the lives of patients via urgent care. In many instances, delivering care in a way that resulted in a life-changing moment for these patients. After fourteen years of service in urgent care, I developed a desire to service patients on a more global scale and be more innovative. So, I began my own business as an urgent care specialist via virtual visits in telemedicine and more specialized care via concierge medicine. As a result of the challenges of my life, I am now the owner of a thriving concierge, direct primary care, and telemedicine practice, who delights in encouraging, empowering, and personalizing healthcare for the busy professionals I service. Due to the services I provide, my patients are more productive, happier, and effective in their personal and professional lives. This allows them to empower others that they touch in their lives, leading to a more productive community, nation, and even the world.

Chapter 1

HEALTH SCREENINGS

"I am a healthy individual, why do I need a health screening?"

Medicine is changing rapidly every day. It is moving and innovative. We are saving lives through technology. We have screenings to help decrease the likelihood of an adverse outcome, disabilities, or death.

While it is definitely your choice to utilize these health screenings, their purpose is solely to help prolong life and prevent unnecessary disability or deaths at earlier ages.

Each year, younger and younger women are diagnosed with breast cancer. Each year, there are deaths as a result of breast cancer at younger ages. Half of the diagnosed cases are preventable. Screening is the only known factor to positively influence outcome regimens. Do you have your monthly breast exam? I encourage you to do it after your monthly cycle to help you remember this task. You are checking for lumps, nipple discharge, unusual appearance of the breast, and any growths exuding from the nipple. Screening is key. If you are forty years old or older, you need an annual mammogram. History of breast surgeries and augmentations may require the need for more specialized imaging if the initial mammogram is abnormal.

The pap smear is used as a screening tool to detect early

cervical cancer. It should be done every three years to evaluate your risk for cervical cancer. There are stages to this disease that if detected early can be treated and save someone's life. Whether sexually active or not, every woman older than twenty-one years old needs a pap smear every three years. At the age of thirty, you may lengthen the pap smear screening plus HPV testing to once every five years. I encourage you to consult with your physician regarding this particular decision. At the age of sixty-five, the pap smears are no longer recommended. However, every woman needs a pelvic exam every year regardless of your age. Pap smears are no longer recommended after age sixty-five due to the risk of cervical cancer being much less at this age.

For men, prostate cancer has also been diagnosed in younger individuals. A simple screening blood test should be performed every year for men over the age of forty or in younger patients that have a family history of the disease.

Every year, young men and women battle colorectal cancer. Many patients will not go in for screening due to "not liking the way the test is run." The screening test for colorectal cancer is a colonoscopy. During this procedure, the patient is placed under anesthesia and a scope with a camera is placed into the rectal area and travels up to your colon. This allows the gastroenterologist to visualize your colon tissue to be sure there are no signs of cancer. He or she may take a sampling of tissue to send to the pathologist to test your cells for any changes indicative of cancer.

Early detection is key in the staging and ultimately the outcome of a colorectal cancer diagnosis.

If your family has a history of diabetes, you need

annual screening for diabetes starting in the year your family member was diagnosed or at age forty, whichever comes first. For individuals who are overweight or obese, screenings should start at age forty and at least once every three years if the results are normal. For individuals with no risk factors, who are not overweight or obese, screenings can start at age forty-five and every three years thereafter assuming the results are normal. This is done by checking a fasting blood glucose—a blood sugar level taken the morning after not eating after midnight the evening before on two separate occasions.

Obtain a yearly fasting cholesterol level. This is a very simple test that yields potentially dramatic results. High cholesterol is one of the five risk factors for stroke and heart attacks. If your cholesterol is elevated, correction of the level via diet and/or medications will help to decrease this risk. This is especially evident with family histories of stroke and myocardial infarction (MI).

With technology of the twenty-first century, we are in the driver's seat with these cancer diagnoses and outcomes. We need to be the driver. Your body loves you, love it back.

ACTION ITEMS

I AM _____ (age).
The following are the screenings I need:

1) _____

2) _____

3) _____

Chapter 2

BENEFITS OF
DRINKING WATER

"Why do I have to drink water? It's nasty . . ."

Almost 70 percent of our body is composed of water when we are born. As adults, water comprises over 60 percent of our body. Almost 75 percent of our muscles are composed of water. Nearly 85 percent of our brains are composed of water. Every single cell in every organ and tissue in your body needs water to function properly. We actually lose two to three liters of water daily with simple life processes, such as urine excretion, defecation, sweating, and even breathing. Water aids in washing out impurities, especially in the kidney. The recommended dose of water is two liters per day for women and three liters per day for men.

Do you love your kidneys? I sure hope so. If you do, you must drink water.

The kidney is the organ in your body that filters your blood and removes waste. Eighty percent of your blood is composed of water. Your kidneys extract the waste from your blood and place it in the urinary tract to be excreted as urine. They are able to retain water via the use of a chemical, called Antidiuretic hormone (ADH), that is released by your brain in the state of dehydration to tell your kidneys to "hold on to the water, we are dehydrated." The organ that is a part of your brain, called the hypothalamus, senses the sodium concentration level in the kidneys to determine whether or not to release the ADH. ADH acts at the site of your kidneys to prevent water loss. So, the first benefit of drinking water is to aid in the balance of your bodily fluids. This is extremely important as we know that all the cells in your body need water to function.

Dehydration can also contribute to the development of kidney stones. If you frequently develop kidney stones, you are at increased risk of developing chronic kidney disease. The second most common reason that patients are seen in primary care clinics is due to urinary tract infections. The number one cause of a urinary tract infection is lack of appropriate water intake.

Your skin needs water to function as well. Would you like to have soft, glowing skin? Adequate water intake is one of the most simple but easy and inexpensive ways to help ensure you have smooth and glowing skin. Acne can actually be exacerbated by decreased water intake. Getting adequate water intake also reduces the likelihood of premature wrinkling. Yes! Water is a weapon against Father Time in so many ways! Let's see how else . . . Water can be helpful in your weight-loss regimen as well. It helps in two different ways. First, if you choose water instead of sugary or high-calorie drinks, your calorie intake will decrease, leading to weight loss. Especially if you are a converter. The process of converting from sugary drinks with every meal to water with every meal is very beneficial for your health and weight loss. In addition, you can even try preloading or drinking eight ounces of water prior to each meal. It will give you the sensation of fullness and you will eat a little less, leading to weight loss. It also decreases the likelihood of overeating. Your thirst center and hunger center are neighbors in your brain. So when you are thirsty you may perceive a hunger sensation when you really are thirsty. (US World Medical Daily, July 2013.) Seventy-five percent of Americans are chronically dehydrated. Being dehydrated has been shown to linked to chronic fatigue, anxiety, memory issues, and joint pain.

Your brain cells need water to function. Water helps to cushion the brain and the spinal cord. So, if you have inadequate hydration, the cells of your brain that communicate with one another may not function properly. This can present you with challenges in thinking and reasoning ability. With dehydration, patients frequently experience slowed thinking and fatigue. Remember, this is partially due to the fact that our brains are composed of 70 percent water as well. The result of dehydration in your nerve cells will be slower communication between each other. This can make you feel as though your brain is "foggy." It can affect your memory and recall. Lack of adequate hydration stresses our brain.

Your gastrointestinal system also needs water. Water plays a vital role in the production of both urine and feces. Without adequate water intake, you can experience abdominal cramping and constipation. The number one cause of constipation is lack of water. You can also get increased acid buildup in the stomach leading to heartburn symptoms. Adequate hydration plays a vital role in the digestion process.

Did you know that water helps to cushion every joint in your body? Your knees, your wrists, your elbows, every joint. There is a cushion-like material in the vertebrae of your spine called cartilage. At least three-fourths of cartilage is made of water. Therefore in individuals that are dehydrated, they can start to have joint or arthritis pain. In patients that have an underlying joint disease, achiness or pain in that joint can be exacerbated by inappropriate water intake.

So, where else is water helpful? It can help boost your exercise performance. In this case, if you are dehydrated and start exercising, after about thirty minutes you will begin to feel fatigued. This is because every cell in your body needs water to help perform. Therefore, adequate water intake will help to boost your exercise performance.

Water helps to regulate body temperature. When you are hot, water moves to the top layer of your skin and is released as sweat. As water moves to the surface layer of skin, it cools the body. This is why it is vital for individuals working outside in extreme warm temperatures to be sure they are hydrating well. Lack of adequate hydration in this environment can lead to heat strokes. This is due to lack of water in the cells to help cool the body temperature.

In addition, water is used in the production of saliva and mucus. Saliva and mucus help with digestion and decrease likelihood of tooth decay. Water also helps to keep our mouth clean.

Lastly, there are four acute situations where water intake has proven to be vital: if you have 1) a fever, 2) nausea, vomiting, or diarrhea, 3) are outside sweating or exercising, or 4) you are spending time outside in hot temperatures.

Although most Americans are aware of the importance of consuming water on a daily basis, most of them do not follow the recommendations and drink at least two liters of water daily for women and three liters for men.

Inevitably, you are in control of your destiny of health and wellness. How much are you willing to invest in yourself? Take the Water Dare: Drink two liters of water every day for one week. Keep reminders in your phone and calendar that will prompt you daily to keep your commitment. Every morning, take a moment to scale yourself as to how tired or rested you feel: zero is completely exhausted, ten is completely rejuvenated. Write in your Vitality Journal each morning and evening how rested or tired you feel. Record any days where you were surprised by a change in energy level. At the end of the week, review your data in your journal. What difference did that week make?

ACTION ITEMS

How much water do you drink daily?

_____

Name three things you learned about water that you did not already know:

1) _____

2) _____

3) _____

What is your daily water goal?

_____

Chapter 3

BENEFITS OF EXERCISE

Here we discuss the importance of exercise and what it can do for your body. Adults need 150 minutes of moderate aerobic exercise activity every week for maximal health benefits. In America, over half of the population does not exercise on a consistent basis.

The number one known benefit of exercise is maintaining weight loss. When you exercise, your metabolism is boosted and you burn calories. However, this concept is practiced best when combined with a dietary change if you are attempting to lose weight. Exercise speeds up your metabolism so that you can go on to burn calories for hours even after you have stopped exercising.

Exercise helps fight the development of a number of chronic disease processes. This includes high blood pressure. Consistent exercise has been shown to help decrease blood pressure. In addition, it can be used to help maintain or in some cases prevent developing high blood pressure in patients with a strong family history of high blood pressure. It also aids in decreasing the risk of a heart attack and stroke through the conditioning of your cardiovascular system and reduction in cholesterol levels. In addition, exercise boosts the production of HDL or high-density lipoproteins—which is your "good cholesterol." It services as a "dump truck" to help remove LDL or low-density lipoproteins ("bad cholesterol") from your system. Also, exercise aids in the delivery of oxygen and nutrients to your organs to help them work more efficiently.

Exercise helps to decrease stress and anxiety. When you exercise, there are endorphins, also known as "happy hormones," which are released that help to elevate your mood. These hormones also act on receptors in your brain to help decrease pain. So when you exercise you feel happier, more relaxed, less anxious, and experience reduced pain.

Exercise has shown to be extremely important in maintaining muscle strength and building strong bone density. Lifting weights in addition to being sure you have a good protein intake is key in building muscle mass. This is very important as we get older, for our bodies naturally lose muscle and bone strength as we age. Examples of natural sources of protein include lean meat, fish, eggs, beans, and nuts.

How can exercise help my sex life?

The practice of consistent cardiovascular conditioning has a direct and lasting effect on your sexual activity in several different ways. First, your heart is better conditioned for sex when you exercise, increasing your stamina. You have more energy and will be less likely to tire out early in your sexual experience. In addition, your blood flow is naturally improved from exercise and this increases blood flow to your sexual organs, improving your sexual function as well. Exercise leads to better strength, flexibility, and stamina.

There is a direct correlation between increasing physical activity during exercise and increasing sexual encounters.

"But Doctor Celeste, I hate exercise. I'm just not an exercise person."

"I hate going to the gym."

"I would love to exercise, but I'm just too busy with these three toddlers."

So, what can you do? You have to find what exercise regimen works for you. Every personality is different. Some people love to be outside, other individuals love to go to the gym, while some just hate exercising by themselves. Many moms and dads have very complex schedules.

NO worries, just find the activity that best suits your personality.

For all you social butterflies, find an exercise class that you can do with a group or with a friend. For instance, step classes, water aerobics, high-intensity workout groups, walking, or spinning classes.

For all you loners, try the gym, bike trails, run the neighborhood, workout tapes, or even buying a piece of gym equipment for your home, like a treadmill or stationary bike. In addition, what also helps is finding your music motivation or playlists that keep you upbeat and moving.

For you busy moms and dads with little ones, try incorporating your workout into an activity that includes the kids—family workouts! Schedule thirty to forty minutes a day at least four days a week for exercise activity with your kids. You can play tag, hide and go seek, walk as a family, or even bicycle to the local park together. In addition, if you have a holiday coming up, try to incorporate exercise into the gathering. For example, for the Fourth of July, you can plan it at a park that will allow you to set up an obstacle course or you could go swimming or play basketball. A good game of basketball is always fun with a family.

Yet another example would be an Exercise Egg Hunt. Find the plastic eggs they have at Easter time and place an exercise activity in each egg. Go hide the eggs. Bring all the children out to find them. As they find an egg, the first person who finds one checks the egg. Everyone does the physical activity found within the egg together—for example, twenty jumping jacks. Then you start over. At the end of an hour, the kids will be happy because you played with them and you will be happy you got in some exercise.

"But Doctor Celeste, I can't jump due to my chronic knee injury!" No problem, do upper body movements instead. You adjust the workout for whatever limitations you may have. Doing an upper body workout can help to condition your heart in much the same way as a total body workout. The activity may not be as intense but you will still get in a great workout.

Another way to get in the exercise is to dance. Turn the music up, sing, and dance with the kids. They will declare you are the best mom or dad in the world. You can also do yardwork as a form of exercise that will aid with cardiac conditioning.

There is an additional invaluable benefit of exercise that is even better for two reasons. Number one, you are getting the exercise you need to condition your heart, maintain your weight, keep your blood pressure lower, and help you maintain a destressed environment while dealing with little ones. Number two, which is just as powerful, you are setting a remarkable example to your son and/or daughter to see how important exercise is at such an early age.

Can you imagine what impact we as adults could make around the country to help address the childhood obesity problem by consistently serving as a role model for how we should exercise regularly and to do it as a family? And what is even better is they are learning from their most influential role model, their parent, that they will be more likely to keep this going in their own life and teach their children the same. Impact.

ACTION ITEMS

What are three ways that you think exercise will personally transform your life?

1) _____

2) _____

3) _____

Chapter 4

HEART MATTERS

"Why does your heart matter so much?"

What is a heart attack? A heart attack occurs when the blood flow to the heart is compromised. The most common way this occurs is from plaque formation, which is a combination of cholesterol and inflammatory substances. When a plaque has formed it subsequently decreases the blood flow in that particular portion of the heart. When there is a decrease in blood flow, there is subsequently a decrease in oxygen to this portion of the heart. This can result in damage to this particular portion of the heart muscle supplied by the blood vessel. This is called a heart attack.

Heart attacks are now occurring more frequently, especially in the last decade, and in younger individuals. A large part of this is attributed to the advances in technology that allow us to do a number of things electronically when they were once done through physical activity. With this adjustment in technology, you must put more effort into ensuring that you get adequate physical activity to fight the risk of heart disease. In addition, the American diet has a reputation for being unhealthy. It matters what we put in our bodies and the length of time we spend with these unhealthy habits. One person's timeframe may be different from someone else's timeframe. Your diet can adversely increase your risk for having a heart attack if it is not heart healthy.

"Why didn't I have a warning that my heart was not doing well?"

The plaque collection that occurs happens slowly over a period of time. Whenever we have a decrease in blood flow to the heart muscle as a result of the plaque, the neighboring blood vessels will naturally reroute themselves to go to that portion of the heart. This occurs in an attempt to help provide the heart muscle that has been compromised with some blood flow. This is the way God made our hearts.

Typically, there are limited strong warning symptoms in patients in the days and weeks leading up to their heart attack. The most common symptom people complain of is chest discomfort. People will describe this in varying ways: I am having chest pain, chest tightness, chest heaviness, and even "I feel like I have an elephant on my chest."

Any of these descriptions of chest discomfort may be heart-related chest pain. However, everyone that has chest pain is not having a heart attack. Knowing these symptoms can be vital so that you may aid yourself or a loved one in seeking an assessment sooner rather than later to differentiate the symptoms they are having.

In addition, these patients may complain of shortness of breath, breaking out in a sweat, having left arm or neck or jaw pain, or even acid reflux symptoms. Others complain of atypical symptoms of dizziness or lightheadedness.

There are patients who have no chest pain at all that are having a heart attack. They may say I feel dizzy and lightheaded and slightly short of breath. The atypical symptoms as previously listed are more common in women than in men for a heart attack.

Any combination of these symptoms is concerning for a patient having a heart attack. It is very important to seek treatment right away.

What do I do if I am having these symptoms? What do you do if you witness someone having these symptoms?

Call 911 right away.

A number of people will hesitate to call 911 because they say they want to wait it out. They want to see if it gets better. Others talk themselves out of calling because they are in denial. "Maybe I am not having a heart attack. I do not want to cause a false alarm."

They tell themselves that they are just tired or restless. Sometimes they may be fearful of what will be found. You need a professional consultation with a physician to determine that. It is better to get the assessment and find out your heart is normal than not checking and you succumb to the damage in your heart that could even lead to death.

Value yourself and the individual, call 911 right away.

The largest predictor for a heart attack is the amount of time that passes between the time of the injury and the time of treatment. There are three possible outcomes when someone has a heart attack. The first is death. You or your loved one can die from a heart attack. Even with all the technological advancement, you can die in 2020 from a heart attack. The second is temporary damage to the heart muscle that can be minimized through the use of stents, which are placed to reinforce the flow of blood of that portion of the heart that suffered temporary lack of blood flow. If the placement of a cardiac stent would not be effective, a bypass of the diseased portion of the blood vessel may be necessary to return the blood flow distal to the blockages. With this outcome, measures are taken to decrease the likelihood of a repeat cardiac event. There are medications to block your heart muscle from reforming itself after a heart attack. This is an event called remodeling, which can happen with changes in the muscle of your heart pumping chamber, called your left ventricle. There are medications to decrease plaque formation through decreasing cholesterol levels. The third outcome is the development of a chronic complication, heart failure. Lack of blood flow can result in the heart muscle tissue dying altogether, resulting in decreased muscle function. This causes a decrease in the amount of blood pumped from that portion of the heart in each beat. This can cause backup of blood flow in the heart, which may manifest itself with swelling of the lower extremities, which is one of the most common symptoms of heart failure.

Decreasing the time between when you have chest pain and when you seek treatment, you reduce the risk of complications from the heart attack, like heart failure.

"What can I do to avoid a heart attack altogether?"

To avoid a heart attack, decrease the risk factors. The five risk factors for heart attack include hypertension, high cholesterol, diabetes, family history of heart attacks, and smoking.

If you have high blood pressure or a family history of high blood pressure, it is key to have regular assessments by your physician, as well as monitoring your blood pressure at home.

"What is blood pressure?"

Blood pressure is the measure of the pressure across a blood vessel wall. High blood pressure means the amount of tension is elevated above normal. Normal blood pressure is 120/80 or less. The top number is your systolic blood pressure, which is the amount of force at which your heart is beating. The bottom number is the diastolic blood pressure, which is the amount of force at which your heart rests. To obtain a diagnosis of high blood pressure you must show consistently elevated readings on at least two separate readings on two separate days. For patients with mild hypertension, which is defined as blood pressure 120–130/80–90, we typically treat it with a healthy diet and exercise. Blood pressure 140/90 or higher is generally treated with blood pressure medications. Each patient is assessed individually pertinent to their family history to determine when is the appropriate time to start blood pressure medication. Most patients follow the above recommendations, but there are no absolutes. Always follow up after being put on medication. The purpose of the follow-up is to be sure that you are not suffering from any side effects through a checkup and lab work. Most laboratory data ordered is to check your kidney function, thyroid function, liver function, and cholesterol. Blood pressure greater than 180/100 is a hypertensive crisis and is considered a medical emergency. If you or a loved one ever has a blood pressure this high, seek medical treatment immediately.

Risk factors for high blood pressure include family history, smoking, high sodium intake, lack of exercise, diabetes, obesity, obstructive sleep apnea, and heavy alcohol use. Heavy alcohol use is defined as more than one drink a day in women and more than two drinks a day in men.

"Doctor Celeste, what can I do myself to help prevent me from developing high blood pressure?"

"Do I have to take this medication for blood pressure? Can't I just exercise to get my blood pressure down? How long do I have to take this medication?"

These are very commonly asked questions. Let's tackle them one by one.

First, get up and get active if you are not already. Yes! It's exercise again! Exercise can help to lower your blood pressure.

Secondly, if you are prescribed high blood pressure medication and your physician recommends that you take it daily, it is important for you to take it. Generally, I recommend that my patients start a low-sodium and low-cholesterol diet if they are not already following one, in addition to taking blood pressure medications, if they cannot be controlled by diet and exercise alone.

Finally, for the majority of patients, once blood pressure medications are started you may need them for your lifetime. Often patients will ask if they can stop the medications after they have been on them for a few months. Only intense lifestyle changes have been shown to allow the patients to come off of the blood pressure medications after starting them. Examples of these transforming lifestyle changes include weight loss of twenty pounds or more, if appropriate for your body size and type. If you are not overweight, the weight loss will not likely play a role in helping to control your blood pressure. A complete 180-degree dietary change is another example. If you are eating a heavy-sodium, high-sugar diet, changing to a low-cholesterol and low-sugar diet can make a huge difference in your outcome.

It is vital to avoid foods that are high in sodium that will largely increase your risk of developing or worsening high blood pressure. High-sodium foods include tomato sauces, potato chips, canned meats, sports drinks, fried foods, and fatty foods. The daily recommended allowance of sodium is less than 1500 mg. Pay attention to product labels. Read it before you eat it.

Have you had your cholesterol checked? Do you have high cholesterol? Do you have a family history of high cholesterol?

The only way to know is to have it checked.

"I would rather not know."

You cannot crawl into a hole and hope you do not have it. If we know you have high cholesterol, we can take measures to help lower your cholesterol. If you do not, you may suffer a complication like a heart attack or stroke. It is important to have a regular assessment with your physician to check your cholesterol levels.

Are you a diabetic? Have you been screened for diabetes? Do you have a family history of diabetes? Diabetes is known as a double risk factor for a heart attack. If you have diabetes you are at increased risk for having a heart attack. Increased blood sugar levels can increase your risk of a heart attack by compromising optimal flow of blood to that portion of heart muscle. If you want to decrease this risk, having optimal control of your blood sugar is vital. Follow a diabetic diet. Uncontrolled blood sugar can cause microscopic damage to your blood vessels over a long period of time. See your physician regularly. Have your bloodwork done every four months to check your Hga1c. This is a laboratory test that gives you an average of what your blood sugar has been over the last sixty to ninety days. For diabetics, we prefer your Hga1c to be less than 7 percent. Optimal blood sugar control has shown to be very effective in preventing complications from diabetes like diabetic eye disease, diabetic neuropathy (nerve disease of the lower extremities), and diabetic kidney disease, which can lead to the need for dialysis. Dialysis is a process where a machine has to filter your kidneys due to them not functioning properly. Typically patients spend three days a week at the dialysis center for five to six hours. Can you imagine spending three days every week of your life attached to a machine to filter your blood to remove impurities and pump the blood back into your body? This adversely affects the quality of life for these patients. Get your blood sugar tested annually if you are not diabetic and more frequently if you have a strong family history. If you are diabetic, be sure one of the first things you do is go to a diabetes education class. In this class, you typically learn how to check your blood sugar, learn the diabetic diet recommendations, speak with a nutritionist, and learn more detailed information regarding the foods to avoid when you are diabetic.

"But Doctor Celeste, I do not like needles. I do not want to check my blood sugar."

If you do not like using needles, I encourage you to conquer that fear. If you do not monitor your blood glucose, you will likely have to learn to use needles, because if your blood sugar is uncontrolled then you will likely end up on insulin. When and if you do, you could end up sticking yourself four to five times a day instead of twice a day to monitor your blood sugar. In addition, diabetes has been shown to lead to erectile dysfunction in men, especially when blood pressure is uncontrolled.

Cigarette smoking has been directly linked to increasing risk of heart attack. Smoking can cause an increase in your blood pressure. It also decreases the oxygen concentration in the blood. The less oxygen available, the less oxygen there is to serve your muscles and tissues.

To reduce your risk of heart disease try using nicotine patches, nicotine gum, or even oral medications to help you stop smoking.

Patients with a known family history of heart disease

are encouraged to obtain regular consultations with their physician. If you have a family history of heart disease, there are certain pieces of information that will be helpful for you to know. Who has "heart disease"? What is the exact component of heart disease—heart attack, stroke, heart failure, arrhythmia? Be sure to ask both parents and grandparents for their health histories. Depending on how the heart disease presented, they could describe a heart attack in one of a few different ways. They may say simply, "I had a heart attack that began with chest pain." They may say, "I felt weak and fatigued so I saw my physician who sent me for testing that came back abnormal. I had blockages and had to get a stent." Oftentimes if you ask this patient if they had a heart attack, they will say, "No." In their mind they did not have a heart attack, they had a blockage. However, the indication is the same. They have coronary artery disease, which is a blockage of your heart blood vessels.

On other occasions, they may say they had a "light heart attack" at some point in the past but they are not sure when. Others may say, "I never had a heart attack but I had to have open heart surgery." Again, this is a patient who did not present with crushing chest pain and shortness of breath to the emergency room, so in their mind they think they did not have a heart attack.

So why is this important? It is important to understand that even if a patient does not present with the symptoms of a classic heart attack, with the typical presentation and subsequent outline of events, this does not mean they don't pose a risk to you as a family member for heart disease.

Giving a full family history is important in order for your physician to completely assess your health risks and mitigate these risks, especially for heart disease. The heart is a complex and intimate organ. Taking the best care of it breeds wellness for your lifetime. It is your investment into your vitality.

ACTION ITEMS

What are the five symptoms of a heart attack?

1) _____

2) _____

3) _____

4) _____

5) _____

What is the first thing to do if you or your loved one starts having chest pain?

_____

Name three ways you will change your life to decrease your risk of heart attack and stroke:

1) _____

2) _____

3) _____

Chapter 5

YES, STRESS CAN KILL YOU! HOW? WHAT DO I DO?

"How do I know if I am stressed?"

Some of the most common physical symptoms of stress include weight gain, acne, insomnia, reduced sex drive, heart attack, stroke, infertility, poor digestion, depression, irregular periods, and hair loss.

Throughout your life, there will always be "stressors" or challenges. What can make a pivotal difference on your health and wellness is how you deal with these stressors. How you channel the stress in your life can affect you physically and, for many, shorten your lifespan as a result of stressors causing negative physical manifestations, such as a heart attack or stroke.

The primary cause of stroke is uncontrolled or fluctuating blood pressure. One of the triggers for elevated blood pressure in many patients is stress. Stress that goes unchecked can lead to prolonged anxiety, which has been shown to lead to poorly controlled blood pressure in hypertensive and cardiac patients. When you have uncontrolled blood pressure over a long period of time, you increase your risk of stroke. When you do not learn positive and effective ways to cope with stress, it can have a profound effect on your blood pressure being increased.

In addition, stress has been shown to contribute to heart attacks. Over a long period of time, stress can have negative effects on your heart. Your heart has to work twice as hard when it is stressed than when it is relaxed. For this reason, one of the issues addressed in the treatment plan of patients who have recently suffered heart attack or stroke is, "What stresses does the patient have in his or her life?"

The purpose of the entire treatment plan for this patient is to prevent another recurrence. Meaning, stress is not just "something you need to get over." It is vital to address the underlying issue(s) causing the stress. If there are work or home stressors, it is best to attempt to change or at the very least adjust the environment(s) to avoid further negative impact from the stressor. There are recent studies that suggest a link between physical illness, stress, and the coping mechanism for stress or the lack thereof.

Uncontrolled stress can also lend itself to the development of major depression. Some can find themselves in an overwhelming, prolonged sad state due to focusing on the stressors. It often is characterized by them feeling as though they are in a loop constantly focusing on the negative aspects of their situations, feeling like it will never improve. Soon, they find themselves lulled into a depression by the constant looping of these negative thoughts in their minds. Chemically, when you are stressed you release a hormone called cortisol, which is known as a "stress hormone." When the body is under a great deal of stress, these cortisol levels increase and serotonin ("happy hormone") levels are decreased. This leads to feelings of depression.

It is noted that stress incurred from a troubling marriage or divorce can definitely contribute to health issues in your life. In many instances, this is unavoidable when dealing with marital issues. In that case, we must consider the filter. Your mental filter tells us how your brain processes information. As soon as you hear information, it is processed through a filter and your brain decides how to process it.

What is paramount is addressing the cause of the stress. Is there a way to change the situation? Is it temporary or permanent? Can they change their environment?

Oftentimes, there is nothing you can personally do to change the stressor. HOWEVER, you can change YOUR PERSPECTIVE. Perspective changes everything. It is vital to know how powerful your outlook on a stressor can be, especially if there are family-related issues. You cannot change your family—it is who God gave you. What you can do is change your perspective. Be sure that you meditate daily prior to coming in touch with the "stressors." Exercise. It releases happy hormones, namely serotonin. Sleep. Make sure you are getting at least eight hours of rest each night. This alone will help to decrease physical stress and prepare you better to deal with mental stressors of your day. Eat a healthy diet. Feed your body foods that make it function well, and avoid fatty and fried foods, which are more likely to cause you physical stress. Manage your time properly. Grant yourself permission to say "No." Many times we place unnecessary stress on ourselves by wearing too many hats. Be ready. Know that it is coming. Know your positive energy space and how to tap into that. Know in advance where you will go when trouble comes. Go to that safe and peaceful place as you remind yourself that the presenting change or issue may be temporary. Minimize your time if possible with the stressors. If you know it is coming, properly lock them in the appropriate box so as to not let it kill you. Stress does kill but it does not have to. Mindset is key for dealing with stress.

ACTION ITEMS

List three areas of stress in your life:

1) _____

2) _____

3) _____

List three ways you will take an active measure to change things or adjust your filter:

1) _____

2) _____

3) _____

Chapter 6

MANAGING KNOWN HEALTH ISSUES—HTN, DM

"I have ___, now what do I do to minimize what is keeping me from living my best life?"

Screenings/Annual Lab Work

If you are a patient challenged with diabetes or hypertension, KNOW YOUR NUMBERS. You should have an assessment with your physician at least once every four months. You need labs checked twice a year for hypertensive patients and three times a year with diabetics, at minimum. Know where you stand with your blood pressure. How well controlled is it? Hypertensive patients should have a blood pressure monitor at home, whose calibration has been checked to ensure accuracy. Monitor your blood pressure regularly, at least two to three times a week. Keep a blood pressure log to share with your physician. This gives a good illustration of how your blood pressure is running.

Do I have high cholesterol? If so do I need medications? Be sure that you are following a low-cholesterol diet with both hypertension and diabetes. All three diagnoses carry increased risk of heart attack and stroke. Keeping a controlled cholesterol level decreases this risk.

If you are a diabetic, are you checking your blood sugar at home? What was your last Hga1c? What should your Hga1c be? When is it time to have it rechecked? Diabetics should check their sugar daily. It is generally recommended that diabetics check their blood sugar two to three times daily, especially if you use insulin. It is important to have your Hga1c checked every four months as recommended to assist with blood sugar control. The desired range of Hga1c is typically less than 7 percent. Having a thorough discussion with your physician concerning this test and ensuring that you understand the test and the results is vital to decreasing the complications and risks from diabetes.

Diet

Diet plays a central role in how well controlled hypertension and diabetes will be. If you do not follow a low-sodium and low-sugar diet, it can and will increase the likelihood of you suffering complications of hypertension and/or diabetes. If you are diabetic, and you eat one dessert every day, it will affect your blood sugar levels both immediately and over a period of time. Ultimately, it can result in your pancreas not functioning as well at an earlier age. When you eat lots of sweet foods as a diabetic, you put more stress on your pancreas, which can affect its ability to produce insulin over the long run. When your pancreas stops working, you cannot make insulin and must take an injectable form of insulin. This is not desirable for most patients, so following the diabetic diet will assist in decreasing the likelihood of this happening.

Exercise

As previously mentioned, exercise is paramount in maintaining cardiac conditioning. Exercise at least four days a week with forty minutes of moderate exercise activities such as running, bicycling, and fast-pace walking. This will help with your blood pressure control, HDL level (good cholesterol), and mood elevation. Exercise also gives you more energy to be productive at home and work. You can combine any number of various activities to get to the 150 minutes of cardiovascular activity recommended each week.

Follow-Up Visits to a Physician

Keep your quarterly visits with your physician. A lot of healthcare today is centered around disease prevention. There are recommended annual health and wellness screenings which help promote disease prevention and care. Some of the traditional laboratory tests performed at annual and follow-up visits include fasting blood glucose, BMI, cholesterol panel and metabolic panel detailing your kidney and liver function

Managing Meds

If you are given medications to control your high blood pressure or diabetes, take them. There are senseless deaths each year resulting from patients not taking medications. Hypertension is called the silent killer because most patients do not get symptoms with an increase in their blood pressure, yet the increased blood pressure is silently damaging their blood vessels, increasing the risk of heart disease, stroke, neuropathy, retinopathy, and even death. Your physician is like the quarterback telling you what play to run. It is up to you to get the football in the endzone. You have to RUN THE PLAY. That means take your medications. Follow the appropriate diet. Exercise. Love your body that loves you.

ACTION ITEMS

List one to three of your medical diagnoses:

1) _____

2) _____

3) _____

What are you doing for each to ensure it remains controlled and stable?

1) _____

2) _____

3) _____

Chapter 7

LET'S TALK SLEEP

Do you snore? When you wake up do you feel you have obtained a full night of rest? Does your family ever complain that you snore so loudly they can hear you in the next room or even throughout the house?

If you answered yes to any of these, there is a chance you could be challenged with Obstructive Sleep Apnea. Apnea is a pause during breathing. This occurs in some patients as they sleep when their airway becomes temporarily, fully, or partially obstructed. When this occurs, your nervous system is triggered, causing some patients to wake up gasping for air and in some cases they break out in a sweat. When the obstruction occurs, there is subsequently a decrease in oxygen concentration and increase in carbon dioxide due to the temporary block of airflow. Carbon dioxide is the respiratory waste product that is typically released from your lungs when you exhale. With this lack of airflow, it can cause stress on your heart which may present with palpitations. This decrease in oxygen flow can result in complications such as a heart attack, a stroke, or heart failure exacerbation. The risks for each of these diseases is increased dramatically with sleep apnea events. Untreated sleep apnea is theorized to increase the risk of heart disease at least quadruple-fold.

These individuals wake up the next morning not

feeling rejuvenated, but instead feel they have not slept all night. They are typically tired and irritable after not having had a true recharge with sleep. Some symptoms patients suffer with sleep apnea include fatigue, daytime sleepiness, muscle aches, memory loss, decreased concentration, headaches, high blood pressure, and obesity.

"My spouse is saying I have sleep apnea. I told her she is a light sleeper and I would know if I stopped breathing. When I wake up I feel fine. There is no way I could have sleep apnea, could I, Doc?"

The first person that typically triggers the sleep apnea assessment and evaluation is the bed partner. When someone is challenged with sleep apnea, they often stop breathing several times during the night. To watch someone have these symptoms can sometimes be very alarming. Snoring is the most common symptom of sleep apnea. Oftentimes, it is discovered during the annual exam when the spouse or partner reveals to the physician that the patient completely stops breathing, or chokes during sleep. However, on occasion a patient could suffer with sleep apnea and not exhibit loud snoring at all. If you are having any sleep issues, such as waking up not feeling completely restored, you, too, may need a sleep study test. This is the reason awareness is key.

If this occurs to you or your loved one, it is imperative that they have a sleep study test. During this sleep study, they will sleep all night in the hospital. They will place monitoring electrodes on your scalp and heart. Monitoring your heart is important to note the cardiac activity that occurs while you are resting. We want to know what rhythm your heart is in when it is going through these respiratory changes or apneic episodes.

The primary treatment for sleep apnea is a CPAP

machine (continuous positive airway pressure). The machine exudes a gentle pressure over the airway that allows it to stay open instead of becoming obstructed. If you have been diagnosed by a physician as having obstructive sleep apnea, and have had a CPAP machine prescribed, I implore you to use it. On occasion, patients will try the machine and it is challenging to become accustomed to it. It may take a while to adjust. At this moment, some patients make a decision that can be critical, to not use the machine. Patients may complain they cannot breathe the correct way or it is too challenging to get used to the tubing. You may need to take your machine in to be checked with the pulmonology department to be sure you are calibrated correctly and are using it properly. It is imperative to utilize the machine once prescribed, as the risk ultimately is death.

Another method used in the treatment of sleep apnea is weight loss. Individuals with obesity are more likely to have sleep apnea. We are seeing more cases of obstructive sleep apnea in children as the obesity crisis continues to worsen. Just like adults, these children are at risk for death if the sleep apnea goes untreated and/or they can suffer a complication like heart attack or stroke. In rare cases, an individual may lose weight, which improves his or her symptoms of sleep apnea. Weight loss is the only reversible treatment for sleep apnea. In other words, if you lose weight, you can improve the sleep apnea and symptoms in some patients.

"So why do I have to treat this sleep apnea? I live alone and no one even hears me when I snore."

Did you know that untreated sleep apnea could cause you to have a heart attack or stroke and pass away in your sleep? When sleep apnea goes untreated, you could suffer with heart failure, stroke, erectile dysfunction, and/or hypertension. There are certain groups of people that are at more risk of having sleep apnea. Risk factors for sleep apnea include having large tonsils, having a thick neck, obesity, hypothyroidism, high blood pressure, insomnia, and alcohol use.

For these aforementioned reasons, it is especially important for an individual known to have heart disease to have their sleep apnea treated. With the known diagnosis of coronary disease, you are at greater risk to have another event (heart attack). Untreated sleep apnea in a heart patient puts more strain on the heart, increasing the likelihood of another event.

"Why do I need more rest? I get a good five hours of sleep without that machine with all those tubes."

"I typically function fine from four to five hours of sleep, why do I even need eight hours of sleep?"

When we have a lack of rest, our bodies do not get the opportunity to recharge properly for the next day of work. Your mind does not get the opportunity to reset. You also put more stress on your heart by lack of adequate sleep.

When you rest, you are rejuvenated and recharged. Your body gets an opportunity to cleanse impurities. You can get a buildup of inflammation without adequate rest. With adequate sleep you get the opportunity to renew your nutrients, therefore you have more energy.

When you have adequate rest, your memory is improved. Studies even suggest you may help prevent cancer through adequate rest. Resting can also help you lose weight.

"How can I naturally improve my sleep?"

There are several natural remedies which help to improve your sleep. Be sure you are practicing good sleep hygiene. Sleep hygiene includes not watching television while lying in bed. Your mind has a hard time turning off because it has become accustomed to another activity in the bed other than rest.

Do not eat in bed. The bed is for sleep and sex only.

Avoid caffeine after twelve p.m. Caffeine is a major deterrent to sleep. It helps to keep you up.

Exercise is also a wonderful component that adds to helping your body relax in the evening.

How well you treat your body will determine how long your vitality lasts. Adequate rest is necessary and essential to living the best life possible in wellness and health.

ACTION ITEMS

What three things can you do to enhance your sleep?

1) _____

2) _____

3) _____

Chapter 8

ALLERGIES

"Why is my nose always running? I do not have allergies."

For years, people have struggled with how to try and address their allergy symptoms. Allergy symptoms present in a variety of ways. On occasion, someone may have a persistent runny nose off and on. They have never had seasonal allergies before. Now each time they go out to mow the lawn, they end up sneezing, coughing, and having nasal congestion.

When your respiratory passageway (which starts at your nose) comes into contact with certain allergens, it triggers the release of histamines. Histamine is the chemical your body releases upon exposure to certain allergens, like pollen. This causes engorgement of respiratory passageways, causing oftentimes sneezing and nasal congestion. The most common symptoms that allergy sufferers have is typically nasal congestion.

Eventually, exposure to an allergen could lead to a sinus infection or exacerbate asthma symptoms.

What can I do to help decrease my allergy symptoms this fall?

- Obtain an air filter.
- Take an oral antihistamine.

- Use nasal antihistamine spray.
- Drink lots of water.
- Keep your windows up if the pollen count is high.
- Make sure you shower after being outside all day. During the day, you come in contact with several allergens. You want to be sure you wash all of the particles of your face, skin, and clothing when you get home. In addition, leave your shoes at the door so as to not track whatever you have been stepping on all day into your bedroom where you will be sleeping.
- If you suffer with severe allergy symptoms, wear a mask when vacuuming or doing yardwork.
- Use a gentle pressure nasal rinse. This helps to push impurities out of your nose.
- Avoid harsh chemicals that will irritate your allergies. Use natural products when possible.
- Decrease allergy symptoms: home improvement, get rid of the cat/dog.

Avoid allergens that trigger your allergy symptoms. For example, if you have a severe allergy to grass do not play in the grass. While initially the reaction you have may be mild, over time, your reaction to the same allergen can worsen. Limiting exposure to known irritants is always recommended to help keep allergy symptoms controlled.

Oftentimes, patients will have a known allergy to dogs or cats or both but still have the animal in the home. "I have always had a dog and it never bothered me before."

There are two explanations:

1) You can have a mild allergy earlier in life that never bothered you or caused noticeable symptoms. You were able to tolerate exposure to that allergen and live a relatively normal life. So, the dog did not bother him until he was twenty years old but at thirty-three years old it is causing a severe reaction and symptoms. Treatment of this patient is much the same: 1) avoid the allergen, or 2) utilize oral antihistamines.

2) It is possible to not be allergic to something at younger age and later in life develop an allergy to that allergen.

Obtain an Allergy Panel

If you do not know what you are allergic to, it may be difficult for you to determine how to stop your allergy symptoms. If you had an allergy panel at fifteen years old and are having difficulty controlling your symptoms now at age twenty-three, then you may have had a change in your allergen panel. You will need to see your physician to have more testing to determine changes, if any, in your allergen panel. Allergen panels are very effective with assisting in the treatment of recurring allergy symptoms. Repeated exposure to an unknown allergen can present as if the patient is sick when they are having allergy flares due to the repeated exposure. Allergies often do change over time, so when necessary, we will repeat the allergy assessment to be sure we are covering the necessary bases in treatment.

What Foods to Avoid If You Have Allergies

If you have moderate to severe seasonal allergies, you may need to avoid spicy foods. Avoid cayenne pepper, red pepper seasoning, Mexican cuisine, and Cajun spices. These foods have higher amounts of histamines, which can make it easier to trigger your allergy flares. They can contribute to having more severe nasal congestion and sneezing.

Avoid wine or beer. The yeast found in beer or wine can cause an increase in histamine production.

Avoid dairy products. Ice cream and milk cause you to have a thicker mucus production, which can irritate the back of your throat that is likely already irritated from sinus drainage.

Avoid tomatoes. Tomatoes are rich in histamines. The proteins that exist in tomatoes cross-react with pollen in such a way that if you were to eat a tomato on a day that there is a high pollen count, you may develop an irritation in your throat. You may also have scratchiness or a tickle in your throat.

Drink green tea. Green tea has a natural antihistamine property to help fight histamine reactions.

Eat tropical fruits like pineapple. They are very high in vitamins B and C. They contain an enzyme called bromelain that helps to decrease sinus congestion in the sinuses.

Eat fatty fish. Omega 3 fatty acids are found in fish like salmon, trout, and tuna. They contain natural antihistamine properties that aid in reducing inflammation in your body.

Allergy sufferers are often frustrated by repetitive visits to the physician every fall and spring season, most notably. Taking some of the aforementioned steps can play a huge role in helping to prevent so many visits, getting better control of allergy symptoms, decreasing the need for repetitive steroid use to help get allergy symptoms under control, and breathing easier with less coughing and sneezing. I strongly encourage the use of natural food sources to help as well. We can use our diets to improve our health challenges and promote ultimate health, wellness, and vitality in our lives.

Celeste Reese Willis, MD

ACTION ITEMS

Name three things you can do this fall to decrease your allergy symptoms:

1) _____

2) _____

3) _____

Name three foods you eat now that you will remove from your diet to help decrease your allergy symptoms:

1) _____

2) _____

3) _____

Chapter 9

MY WHOLE FAMILY IS SICK! HELP?—FAMILY HISTORY

"Why does my doctor need to know about my family? I want her to take care of me."

Your family health history is paramount in learning the ideal way to live the BEST of your life with optimal health and wellness. The risks of your health history are directly related to the health history of your mother, her parents, and her entire family's history, as well as the history of your father, his parents, and his entire family's history.

For example, let's say your father has high blood pressure, and his father had high blood pressure and heart disease. Your mother has a history of anemia and colon cancer. Her mother has history of diabetes, asthma, and colon cancer, diagnosed when she was forty years old. Your pertinent risk factors include hypertension, colon cancer, asthma, heart disease, and anemia. This means your chances of developing high blood pressure is increased and it is important for you to monitor your blood pressure on a regular basis. I advise the use of a blood pressure cuff for monitoring at home and even at work, especially if it is a stressful environment. In addition, obtaining a fasting cholesterol panel every year will be important as well to be sure to address any changes in cholesterol levels. Be sure to follow up after the labs are drawn to ensure the results are normal or they may need to be addressed. These measures will help to decrease the likelihood of you developing heart disease.

At the age of thirty-five, you will need to start your colorectal cancer screenings due to your family history of colorectal cancer at age forty.

The typical age to start the colorectal screenings is fifty. There is a large genetic component to the development of colorectal cancer. Studies have shown a better outcome for earlier screening in patients with family history.

There are measures you can take that have been shown to deter the development of disease processes. You can exercise and follow a low-sodium diet to aid in the prevention of hypertension. You can follow a low-carbohydrate diet to help prevent the development of diabetes.

"My dad smoked and was an alcoholic—his history does not apply to me, right?"

"I do not smoke. I do not drink. I exercise four days a week. I follow a low-cholesterol diet. My father had a four-vessel open heart surgery at forty years old. I am thirty-seven years old. I figured if I work out and don't smoke I will be fine."

Two issues with these synopses:

1) Your father's medical history is still your family history and therefore you are still at risk for heart disease. He had elevated cholesterol. Even in patients who follow a low-cholesterol diet, if you have a family history of high cholesterol, you are not always able to make dietary changes that can alter the high cholesterol. It depends on how severe the cholesterol elevation is. This is why screenings are so crucial. Nonetheless, any

changes to the diet will help decrease the risk of you having a complication, like a heart attack or stroke.

There have been patients as young as twenty-four years old that have succumbed to a heart attack due to their family history.

2) Even though you work out four days a week, you are still at risk for having high cholesterol and a heart attack. The exercise will definitely help to decrease the risk but it does not mitigate the risk in its entirety.

In summary, your family history serves as a grid to determine what is the best approach to preventative strategies in regard to the disease processes that you are at risk for.

Common Genetic-Linked Disorders: DM/Colon Cancer/Stroke/HTN/Heart Attacks

There are certain diseases that have been known to be genetically linked. These include but are not limited to hypertension, diabetes, colon cancer, stroke, heart attacks, autoimmune diseases, and thyroid disease.

It is always important to be familiar with your family history. How would you like hypertension set loose in your life? Did your mother or father acquire heart disease at a young age? Are you concerned this could happen to you?

If I may be transparent, I witnessed my mother battle with heart disease during my first year of medical school. This had a pivotal impact on my life, personally and professionally. First, I became intense about supporting my mom—reminding her of doctor's appointments, necessary screenings, and the need for consistent exercise. I wanted to use whatever knowledge I had, which was limited as a first-year medical student, to help empower my mother to beat a second heart attack or blockage. I am quite sure I got on her nerves with it. I probably still do, but she's my mom. Secondly, it impacted me professionally. I will never stop fighting to prevent illness and disease in my mom, family, friends, patients, and even the world. I am a voice. I have a mission. I am serving in my purpose. I am a conduit used to help prevent disease and advocate for the ultimate health and vitality in my patients, my family, my friends, and anyone within earshot who wants to live a life of wellness.

My mother's challenge empowered me personally. When I thought of my future, I was determined to prevent the development of heart disease in myself. Determined to beat high cholesterol. Determined to remain vital, healthy, and strong. And so far, God has been gracious in keeping me there. He has blessed me to remain, educate the masses, and be a role model. This is my purpose and my passion.

ACTION ITEMS

Name five disease processes that you have a family history of:

1) _____

2) _____

3) _____

4) _____

5) _____

Chapter 10

I WILL *NOT* GET THE FLU THIS YEAR!

"My eight-year-old child's school class is swapping influenza around like they trade toys."

Sound familiar?

"Every year I get the flu, whether my children manifest symptoms or not."

"I went to my primary physician and they told me to get the flu vaccine. But they did not share anything else as to how I can avoid it."

"EVERY year this flu costs me at least $4,000 in lost work and at least $200 in clinic visits and medication costs. One year it cost me double because I got the flu twice."

The healthcare costs affiliated with the influenza virus are impressive as they rise into the millions annually in the United States. It is especially disparaging during intense flu seasons.

To take or not to take?

There are numerous controversial views on the influenza vaccine. Most physicians recommend it. What is it? The flu vaccine is a small amount of the flu viral antigen. It is just enough to allow your immune system to build up immunity or antibodies which will help you fight the flu when you come in contact with the virus during flu season. The antibodies produced help fight off the flu. Most patients that receive the flu vaccine rarely get the flu virus. If they should happen to have intense exposure and contract the illness, they have extremely mild symptoms compared to their counterparts that did not receive the vaccine. In addition, individuals who had the flu vaccine but succumbed to the flu will typically bounce back sooner from the infection than those who were not vaccinated.

We typically recommend the flu vaccine for two reasons. The main reason is to decrease the likelihood that you will contract the flu. The second reason is to try to prevent the spread of the flu to someone else. The more circulating antibodies you have, the more in your health army artillery to help you fight off the flu virus. Nonetheless, there are certain groups of patients that have a more challenging time fighting off the flu and succumbing to its complications of pneumonia, organ failure, and even death. This includes the elderly and patients with diabetes, asthma, heart disease, and autoimmune disease.

If you think you are experiencing symptoms of the flu, consult your physician for an evaluation immediately.

Is it my allergies or is it the flu?

Are you having flu or allergy symptoms? The symptoms can be challenging to differentiate. Allergy symptoms include sneezing, runny nose, cough, and watery eyes. Flu symptoms include the abrupt onset of headache, body aches, fever, chills, fatigue, runny nose, and cough.

One of the biggest differentiating factors is that the flu is typically characterized by fever, aches, and chills. Allergy symptoms never typically include these.

Allergy symptoms usually are very gradual in onset. Most patients with the flu have a fever. However, just because you do not have a fever does NOT mean you do not have the flu. You can get a sore throat and congestion with either the flu or with allergy symptoms. Chest congestion is very rarely seen with seasonal allergies, but can be a complication of having the flu. In particular, I encourage you to pay attention to the season to give more indication of whether you are having true flu symptoms or are having an allergy flare. Both of these conditions can lead to serious complications if left untreated.

What can I do in my home to prevent the flu?

If one of your children happens to contract the flu, you can take measures to prevent it from spreading to yourself and the rest of your family. First, quarantine the child as much as possible (without alienation).

One of the most basic things you can do to prevent the spread of the flu is simple handwashing with warm water and soap for at least twenty seconds each time. You may also use alcohol hand sanitizer when the use of warm soap and water is not possible.

Utilize antibacterial and antiviral disinfectant spray in each of the rooms daily, especially in his or her bedroom. Use antibacterial and antiviral cleansing wipes to clean all surfaces in your kitchen, living room, and common areas. Wash bed linens and towels frequently. Be sure to wipe down all of your personal devices like cell phones, tablets, and mp3 players to prevent the spread of the antigen. Change your toothbrush on the day of diagnosis and again when finished with medications, if applicable.

In the workplace, we also recommend the use of disinfectant spray and cleansing as well, especially on commonly shared surfaces.

Cough and/or sneeze into your elbow or sleeve to prevent spreading the antigen released when you cough or sneeze.

What are other things I can do to help fight the flu?

There are certain foods that may actually impact how

well we fight the flu. The first is water. Water hydrates every cell in your body, increasing its effectiveness. Drink plenty of water. Get plenty of rest. When you are tired and fatigued, your immune system is down, making it easier for you to contract infections. Take a daily multivitamin. In addition, I personally recommend utilizing some natural food sources to help.

Five Foods to Help You Fight the Flu

1) Pomegranate juice

Pomegranates are a fruit that is full of vitamins and antioxidants via the seeds of the fruit! Antioxidants are very crucial to aid in keeping the cells in your body healthy and to enable you to fight off viruses, keeping down inflammation and preventing liver damage.

They also aid in keeping cholesterol levels down and with symptoms of arthritis. Pomegranate juice has a greater potency of antioxidant activity than green tea, red wine, concord grape juice, cranberry juice, and orange juice. Pomegranate is also a great source of vitamin C and potassium.

2) Elderberry

For over a hundred years, Native and European Americans have used elderberry for its immune support properties. Often given when persons are sick, elderberry has wonderful antioxidant and energy-boosting properties. It can aid in fighting off a cold, the flu, or respiratory infections. Most often elderberry can be found in natural food stores as lozenges, syrup, or capsules.

The elderberry is the fruit of the Sambucus tree. The pure elderberry fruit is poisonous and so it should only be ingested in the form of lozenges, syrup, or capsules.

The elderberry contains many nutrients and vitamins, which include folate, vitamin A, vitamin C, potassium, calcium, and iron. There have been studies regarding the effect of elderberry and its immune-boosting properties.

A study from 2010 showed that persons with flu symptoms who used the elderberry reported less symptoms of fever, headache, and body aches after taking the elderberry for only forty-eight hours.

In addition, elderberry is a wonderful source of fiber, helping to improve symptoms of constipation, reduce blood pressure, decrease cholesterol, and protect against colon cancer and against cardiovascular disease.

3) Cauliflower

Cauliflower is a cruciferous vegetable. It is very rich in antioxidants and vitamins that give your immune system a boost. They also contain choline, an essential nutrient to maintaining optimal health, as it is vital for brain development, liver function, metabolism, and healthy nervous system function. It also supports a healthy gastrointestinal system, as it serves as a barrier to keep bacteria confined to your colon and not in the intra-abdominal area.

Cauliflower is especially beneficial when you are sick, as it contains glutathione, a strong antioxidant that helps you fight off infection.

4) Garlic

Garlic is tasty and a wonderful seasoning for your

culinary delights. We use it to season meats, vegetables, sauces, and a host of other foods. In addition, garlic has very intense immune-boosting properties. It also reduces the risk of cardiovascular disease and improves mental health. It is noted to slow hardening of the arteries and lower blood pressure.

It is a wonderful addition to your diet to aid you in fighting off the flu.

Garlic contains a nutrient called allici, which turns into allicin when garlic is crushed or chewed. This substance contains sulfur and has been shown to boost the white blood cell response (the disease-fighting response) when they encounter bacteria and viruses. Garlic has been shown in several studies to have antibacterial and antiviral properties.

Studies have shown that persons who take garlic supplements have a noticeably less chance of getting a cold or the flu. In addition, for those persons who are taking garlic and have a cold, their symptoms are much less intense and for shorter periods of time. Garlic helps you to recover faster if you have the flu. It is best to consume raw garlic or aged garlic extract for maximum benefits of its usage.

5) Sweet potatoes

Sweet potatoes are root vegetables, which are rich in minerals and nutrients. They are one of the largest natural sources of beta carotene, which transforms into vitamin A in your body. It contains not only large amounts of vitamin A but also vitamin B6 and vitamin C and is packed full of antioxidants. Vitamin A helps to boost your immune system as well as decrease risks of various illnesses, helping you maintain healthy mucus membranes. Low levels of vitamin A have been linked to having decreased immunity.

Sweet potatoes are also great for your digestive system, as they are high in fiber and help to decrease symptoms of constipation. They also help keep the lining of your gastrointestinal symptoms healthy, which is important, as your gut is exposed to disease-causing pathogens as well. Add sweet potatoes to your diet to help you fight off the flu.

You do NOT have to contract the flu this year. Make up your mind now that you will live a life of health and wellness this entire year. Take the following steps to help make that happen:

1) Get your flu vaccine.
2) Charge up your diet with natural food sources to give your immune system a boost.
3) Take care of your daily body maintenance with 150 minutes minimum of cardiovascular activity each week, drink at least two liters of water daily (three liters for men), and take a daily multivitamin.

With these simple steps, you will promote within yourself the ultimate health, wellness, and vitality.

ACTION ITEMS

Name three symptoms of the flu:

1) _____

2) _____

3) _____

Name three things you will institute this year to prevent you from getting the flu:

1) _____

2) _____

3) _____

Name three foods you will start adding to your diet today to help build your immune system:

1) _____

2) _____

3) _____

Chapter 11

IMPORTANCE OF FAMILY TIME AND SELF-CARE

If you truly want to live your best life, enjoy your family. When things are right at home, it decreases stress. You are happier. You are more fulfilled. It is vital as a parent, spouse, and partner to be sure to take time for yourself and your family. You should make noticeable efforts to ensure the security of your family. Most people that schedule family time are less stressed and tend to be in better health than people who do not. Why is this?

"How can we find time together I work two jobs?"

The best way to find time to spend with your family is to schedule family-oriented activities. Cook a meal together. You have to cook dinner anyway. Everyone has to eat. The dinner table is a perfect way to reflect on the day and share in the lives of your spouse and children. Give them the opportunity to know what is going on in your day as well. You will remain in tune with what is happening in everyone's daily life.

You know you want to continue to exercise four days a week. Plan for the family to ride their bikes to go get ice cream after dinner. Multitask. Wear your workout clothing when you drop off your son to football or basketball practice. You can run or walk laps around the field while he practices. Or better yet, you can climb the stairs in the bleachers. You can even form a workout group with the other parents to serve as a role model for your children.

There are several positive effects from family time. Let's review a few of these. Researchers suggest that children who come from homes wherein family time is routinely practiced have better academic performance. Children want to have your attention and typically perform better if they know you are committed or watching. Children who have family time have fewer behavioral issues and less violence in their lives. It is vital for children to have your help and guidance, knowing that you value education. This is reiterated with family time activities, especially dinner time wherein you can review the tasks the child has for the upcoming week such as projects or tests.

When you schedule family time, you strengthen the family bond. When a family plays together, cooks together, and exercises together, they spend time with the family core activities, strengthening the family bond. This is one of the biggest benefits of structured family time.

All of these things lend themselves toward contributing to your family bonding time.

You know what else is vital to strengthening the family unit? You. Everyone needs to be sure to practice adequate self-care.

Are you listening to your body?

It is important to listen to the clues your body is giving you. If you are tired, be sure to rest. If you are thirsty, be sure you drink water. If you are dizzy or have a headache, check your blood pressure and heart rate. Review your most immediate diet. Have you been eating properly? Have you been adequately hydrating yourself? If you are having chest pain, see a physician for further evaluation.

Self-care. What is this and why do I need this? Your body loves you, love it back.

Studies have shown that you need to schedule your self-care time. People who schedule self-care time have less stress, are more productive, and lead happier lives.

What does self-care scheduling mean? Those are days you schedule just for you to take care of all of your personal needs.

Schedule your dental cleaning. Obtain your annual mammogram. Have a woman's exam once a year. Schedule your manicure and pedicure. Go to lunch with friends. Take a vacation at least twice a year. If you cannot leave town, make it a point to have a "stay-cation"—a vacation in your home city in the hotel. Make scheduled time to spend with your spouse. It is very important to nourish your marriage and deepen your bond by your couple "shared" self-care time. Schedule and complete your meditation time every day. Make scheduled time with your children and extended family.

So, with this ladies and gentlemen, I bid you adieu. I will leave you with this. In life, we learn that if your house is destroyed in a tornado, you can replace your house. If you lose your job, you can get another job. If all of your clothing is destroyed in a house fire, you can replace your clothing. If you destroy the one body God gave you, you cannot get another one. Your body loves you. What an impeccable creation the human body is. The way it naturally leans toward repairing itself after all of the things we put our body through. Condition your body. Hydrate it. Nourish it. Protect it. Invest in it. I think your body is worth it. Your body loves you, love it back.

ACKNOWLEDGMENTS

This book would never have been possible without the individuals listed below:

First, thank you to my patients. Thank you for taking this journey with me. Thank you for being a great patient and investing in your own health. Thank you for entrusting me to be the vessel you utilize as you travel to a lifetime of health and wellness. Thank you for entrusting your lives to me. Thank you for believing in me and the brand that is continuously being created and remodeled. Thank you for your loyal following and support of me. Thank you for providing me with the opportunities to care for you and your loved ones, increasing my experience, filling my purpose, and allowing me to operate in my purpose. Thank you for investing in yourself and in your health. I pray these principles are helpful to you as you keep growing, seeking, and pushing your way to improved health.

Thank you to Dr. Draion Burch. Thank you for creating Medical Moguls. Thank you for being selfless and sharing your genius with us. From you I have learned how to utilize my intellectual property to affect the lives of others on a global scale, while serving in my purpose. I sincerely appreciate all you have done, all you are doing, and all you continue to do for us (#MMA20). You have created an indelible mark on my life and career, and for that I am forever grateful. May your arms be filled with blessings so wide, you do not have room enough to receive them.

ABOUT THE AUTHOR

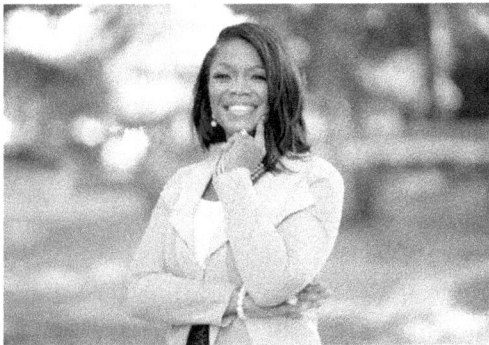

As one of the leading experts in urgent care, Celeste Reese Willis, MD (a.k.a. Doctor Celeste, MD), is a board-certified family medical physician. She is a nationally recognized speaker and consultant whose passion centers around empowering her patients and providing them with excellence in healthcare. In addition, she is a sought-after media expert regarding seasonal allergies, influenza, and hypertension treatment and prevention. Dr. Celeste consistently educates her patients via her online TV show and personalized concierge medical visits. In addition, she provides her patients the opportunity for virtual medical visits for acute health care needs.

With fourteen years of experience in urgent care, with one of the nation's largest urgent care companies, Dr. Celeste has become one of the leading experts and sought-after physicians in her community of Birmingham, Alabama, as well as her state. As a compassionate physician who prides herself on providing patients thorough yet practical healthcare, Dr. Celeste's reputation of providing persistent excellence in healthcare has earned her the title of one of America's favorite urgent care physicians. She earned her medical doctorate at Wright State University School of Medicine in Dayton, Ohio, followed by her residency training at Carraway Hospital in Birmingham, Alabama. Dr. Celeste began moonlighting in urgent care during her second year of residency, where her love of urgent care began.

Being able to solve acute, urgent care needs in varying medical situations grew a further passion of service in medicine. One of her greatest passions is mentoring young girls to pursue their dreams despite the challenges one is presented in life. Dr. Celeste shares her medical knowledge passionately and transparently via her YouTube channel, "Let's Chat with Doctor Celeste, MD." With her experience, love of humanity, compassion, calm but loving bedside manner, and passion about educating her patients in medicine, it is no wonder Dr. Celeste has become America's Favorite Urgent Care Physician.

www.ingramcontent.com/pod-product-compliance
Lightning Source LLC
Chambersburg PA
CBHW051037030426
42336CB00015B/2915